The Chronicles of Phill
(How to Cope With a Neurological Disorder I Got From My Other Two Books)

By Dr. Philip Oldfield

Dedication

I would like to dedicate this book to anyone who is suffering from any progressive neurological disorder, and for their families who are quietly suffering with them. Also, for the volunteers and workers providing the much needed information and support. Especially The Multiple Sclerosis Society of Canada, and The CJD Foundation in the USA.

Table of Contents

Chapters

Introduction

This is the story of Philly Raccoon, in search for answers, getting into mischief, and teaching us all in the process. As patients we need to know the truth, even if the answer is, "I don't know". Approximately two years ago I was acting in a Christmas Pantomime "Puss in Boots" at the Hudson Village Theatre at the age of 56 dancing on stage to Michael Jackson`s "Beat it" along with 15 other people. Now I can only walk with a cane, even then not properly, and my speech at times can get a bit slurred as if I'm drunk, except that my mind is perfectly fine, at least for now. This means of course that I can remember everything that has happened (so embarrassing). I also feel sad when I think about the things I can't do anymore.

A little over a year ago I was told that I had cerebella ataxia. I have had lots of tests done, but so far the cause has not yet been identified, and I believe it's getting worse. Like most people, I suppose my thoughts are somewhat "dark", and I only had two questions for the medical profession to answer, mainly to plan my holidays:

1. What have I got?
2. How long have I got?

When it comes to neurological disorders I do realize that it is extremely difficult to come to a diagnosis, especially in the early stages, and fully understand how difficult it must be for the neurologist. Fortunately for me I had already published a couple of books, the concepts of which has helped me to cope. Both of these are available:

1. Everything I know about stress management I got from Elijah.
2. Everything I know about self-esteem I got from Gehazi.

In this book, I have put together some stories from the patient's view-point. I was getting so frustrated with all that was going on that I started writing about some of my experiences on Facebook (FB); the patient however was not me but Philly Raccoon. I found that by expressing my sense of humor into the situation, that it was actually therapeutic for me. After a few stories, some responses, and my wife Helen telling me to stop putting these up on FB. She was also asking me questions like, "how long have you been in the house?" Helen was obviously getting worried, so I stopped, and then got lots of other people contacting me wanting to hear more Philly Raccoon stories. So by popular demand here they are, a work of creative non-fiction in which the medical facts are correct as well as the dialog as far as I know, apart from the obvious "raccoon specific items" e.g. using ones tooties for checking the doctors reflexes, and obviously the last two stories about the Walk to Bethlehem play, which by the way is worth seeing. This is the story so far from the patient's perspective. I still don't know what I've got, but I do know that ataxia doesn't have many good outcomes. However, after being refused a request to have a 14-3-3 test (just for my own peace of mind), and please note that all the other tests were negative; I had decided to revisit the events leading up to the Bovine Spongiform Encephalopathy (BSE) commonly known as Mad Cow disease outbreak in the UK (Yep! I was living there at the time), and cases of Creutzfeldt – Jakob disease being observed now. I came up with some very interesting idea's and points to consider. Philly Raccoon has also come up with an idea for a possible cure; he's hoping to get the prestigious "Big Plate Foodies Prize" for Physiology or Medicine. I would certainly like to know what the rest of the scientific community think of it.

About the author

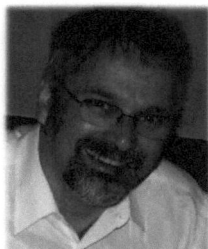

Dr Philip R. Oldfield started his scientific career in 1974 in the Clinical Biochemistry Department at the Royal Postgraduate Medical School, Hammersmith Hospital London, England. Since then he has obtained three degrees; including a D.Phil obtained in 1982. The subject of his research was "Proteolytic Control and Rheumatoid Disease". In 1986 he was given the Baker Award for his work on Digoxin-Like-Immunoreactive-Substances. He has over 30 years experience in service to the pharmaceutical and biopharmaceutical industry specializing in ligand binding assay techniques including hybridization assays. He is currently President and CEO of his own consulting company. Dr Oldfield has a keen interest in forensic science and is an Associate Member of the Royal College of Pathologists, a Fellow of the Royal Society of Chemistry, and an active Member of the American Association of Pharmaceutical Scientists. In addition he likes to maintain a link with the local universities, and has been involved in supervising postgraduate students, as well being an occasional guest lecturer. He is currently involved as a committee member to organize symposia and workshops as part of the Drug Development Training Program at the University of McGill.

Philly Raccoon goes for a run

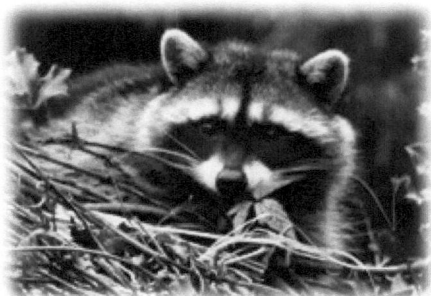

It was the autumn of 2013 and Philly went for walkies (walk) with Helen around the block because she wanted Philly to get his exercise. All started well until Helen started to run, Philly Raccoon not being one to be left behind ran to overtake and at that point realised that his paws refused to take orders. He was kind of running, but more like an out of control "Zombie Raccoon" and almost fell into a ditch. Philly was scared, really scared, nothing like this has ever happened to him before; he heard all about zombies and was hoping that he wasn't going to turn into one. Philly called out to Helen, "Stop! Stop!" there's something wrong with me. Philly explained everything to Helen. Helen then took his paw and they walked back home together.

Philly was not a happy raccoon that night, and decided to go and see the doctor. In the town of Hudson it takes at least a month from the time one books an appointment to actually seeing someone in person. Finally the day came and Philly presented himself to the Doctor who keeps on telling him to eat healthy food (foodies) instead of the crap he gets from garbage cans. She also asked him what is wrong and Philly said:

"Doctor! I'm not happy!" The Doctor then took notice because Philly is usually a very happy raccoon, she asked him to walk up and down the hallway, and then to walk with one paw just in front of the other, like lady raccoons do, at which point he fell over. She said: "You have ataxia, and have to see a neurologist." She explained that ataxia is when you walk and run funny (zombie-like), and it can have many causes. Philly Raccoon needed to get some blood and wee wee tests done. First the blood had to be taken, it took some doing but they managed to get some in the end, (Philly also took blood). Wee wee samples were easier to obtain, Philly was happy to give them lots of wee wee, (but not all of it in the container). Philly then asked the laboratory staff if they needed any poo poo samples, and they all shouted Noooo! However, after all these efforts the results came back negative.

Next step see the Neurologist.
<u>Questions:</u>
1. **What should Helen have done before walking back home?**

2. **The blood and urine tests were the fairly routine ones, but she also asked for "Anti-Nuclear Antibodies" which was normal, and "Vitamin B12" which was above the upper limit of normal. Comment on what this could mean and whether or not it could explain Philly's symptoms?**

3. **Explain the term "Ataxia" and list possible causes?**

Philly Raccoon sees the Neurologist

Philly was very fortunate because he could chose who he could see. There was this lady neurologist; however, when Philly looked her up on the internet her rating wasn't very good with comments like: "she wasn't very nice, and the receptionist was even worse." Fortunately, Helen told Philly that he was already a patient of a very good neurologist so he went to see him. An appointment was made, and Philly presented himself at the doctor's office in Pointe Claire at the appointed time. Philly Raccoon was hit with a hammer (Philly didn't like that), made to walk up and down, and then to walk with one paw just in front of the other, like lady raccoons do, he fell over again. The neurologist said that he had dystonia in his right paw, confirmed that he's got ataxia, and that he needed more blood and wee wee tests done. The staff in the laboratory drew lots to see who would be the one to take the samples. Philly had no idea that he was so popular, they even had to resort to drawing lots to determine who the lucky person would be. Philly was so overwhelmed and wanted to show his appreciation that he gave them poo poo samples as well. However, all these tests including the Magnetic Resonance Imaging (MRI) came back negative too. So in the end the neurologist told Philly that there was nothing else he could do, and referred him to the specialists at the hospital.

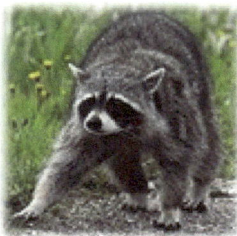

[Ataxic gait]
**Philly Raccoon waits to get summoned to the hospital.
and waits!
and waits!
Until the Neurologist got so feed up that he contacted the hospital directly!**

Questions:
4. Why did the Neurologist hit Philly with a Hammer; what was he assessing and why?

5. Explain the term "Dystonia"?

6. Why did the Neurologist ask for the following tests to be done?

   a. Complete Blood Count (CBC) with peripheral smear

   b. Alanine Aminotransferase (ALT)

   c. Ceruloplasmin level

   d. Erythrocyte Sedimentation Rate (ESR)

   e. Vitamin E level

f. Anti-cardiolipin antibodies (ACA)

g. 24 Hour urinary copper

Philly Raccoon goes to hospital

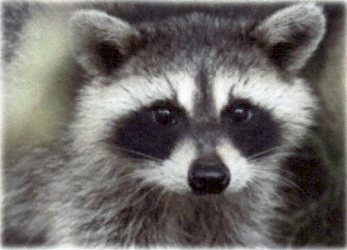

Philly Raccoon was summoned to the Montreal General Hospitals Neurological Unit for an examination. Philly being a very clever raccoon didn't bother to revise. When he got there, the doctor told him to relax after which he hit him with a hammer. Philly Raccoon said: "how can I relax when you hit me?" The doctor explained that he needed to look at reflexes, at which point Philly Raccoon used his tooties (teeth) to check the doctor's reflexes. After over two hours three doctors came to look at him. The chief doctor called the consultant told Philly that his brain was crossed-wired and needed to see a personal trainer to teach him how to walk and run again. Philly Raccoon did not understand how someone like Kruger could help him and asked what would cause such a thing? The consultant said that stress can cause that, but how could that be? Philly had written a book on stress management, and besides how can stress make you run and walk funny without any other stress symptoms? The consultant then asked Philly if anything catastrophic had happen in his life recently. Oh! Oh, said Philly, it can't be, could it, now I remember, and Philly Raccoon proceeded to tell them an untruth about the time that he was abducted by aliens who took the brain out to study; he told them that he felt light headed and there was this experience like a floating sensation. At that point Philly was wondering (out loud) if they put it back in right, if not, that would explain being crossed-wired. The doctor who hit Philly with the hammer started laughing very loudly, and got a look from the consultant that could only be followed by spontaneous combustion of the recipient. The doctor then asked Philly if he could have a copy of his book, and Philly said yes. The consultant then turned on Philly and said very loudly what do you expect me to do? Philly asked respectfully, if it would be possible to have a 14-3-3 test and an EEG please. The consultant said that the 14-3-3 test would have to be sent to a special place in Winnipeg and that Philly's name would have to go on some sort of black-list, and also said that the result would more likely come back as a false positive making Philly panic. In the end the consultant refused and instead booked him for another MRI. Philly then had to see the very nice receptionist to get another appointment. She likes Philly, especially after what he said to the doctor's; she also diagnosed Philly as having Obsessive Compulsive Disorder (OCD). What makes you think that Philly asked? The very nice receptionist replied "**You are tidying my desk**" but don't worry, although that too is neurological, it's another department.

The diagnosis is currently: **Divergent........**
Philly Raccoon still needs to have more tests done, this time he'd better revise.

Questions:

7. **Why did the consultant suggest that Philly was "crossed-wired"?**

8. **Can stress be responsible for Philly Raccoon's symptoms?**

9. Was the consultant right in saying that Philly ort to see a personal trainer?

10. What was on Philly's mind when he asked for a "14-3-3 test" and an "electroencephalo-gram" (EEG)?

11. What does the consultant think he's got?

12. What do you think the "Black list" that the consultant referred to is (Philly was already upset because he was tested for anti-cardio-lipin antibodies)?

13. List all of the medical conditions that Philly knows he hasn't got?

FB comments from a friend:
Got a note from Tanya Watanabe "I'm hopeful for a happy ending to the Philly Raccoon's story!! Always thinking about you and admire your positive energy!!" And "Thought of you when I saw this at Comic-con!!"

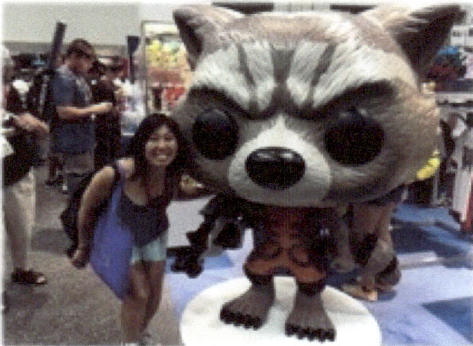

Philly replied "Thank you Tanya and I miss you!"

Philly Raccoon has an MRI

Philly Raccoon was summoned yet again to the Montreal General Hospital, this time for an MRI. Philly was told that he had to fast; WHAT! Fast? Philly being a little raccoon didn't know what fasting was because they like to be surrounded by foodies, and besides it was the brain that was going to be MRIed not his tummy. Anyway, when Philly Raccoon got there he was asked when he had his last one done. Six months ago said Philly. The nice lady then replied then why are you having one done now, so soon. I don't know said Philly, I wanted a 14-3-3 test and an EEG, but they wouldn't listen to me. That seemed to have ended the conversation. The nice lady then put an IV into his arm. Philly said ouch! What's that for (ready to bite)? Now the not so nice lady said she was going to inject a silver metal called Gadolinium. Philly had heard about this having seen "X-Men". Oooo! Philly had thoughts of retractable metal claws (he saw them on television), claws that can cut through metal garbage cans ... Yes!

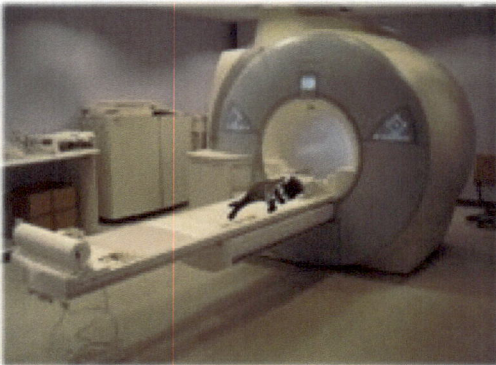

Philly Raccoon was then led into a room where there was a huge garbage can on its side and made to go into it. It took some doing, but they did it in the end, with the help of a tranquilizer gun and a roll of duck tape. Philly heard lots of noise, but fell into a deep, deep sleep, dreaming of those retractable claws. After the noise stopped Philly Raccoon was told that he could go.

Several weeks had past and still no retractable metal claws, but he still dreams of getting them!
<u>Questions:</u>

14. **Why did Philly have an MRI so soon, and do you consider that was the best course of action?**

15. **Why was gadolinium used in this procedure?**

16. **Now what do you think the consultant was thinking?**

17. **What needs to be assessed in Philly prior to administering gadolinium, and describe the medical condition associated with gadolinium toxicity (Hint: it's not retractable metal claws)?**

<u>FB comments from a friend:</u>
Philly got a note from Marion Saunders saying "I hope Philly Raccoon is quite recovered from the ordeal!"
Philly replied "No raccoons were injured during the procedure. As for people, well that's another matter. I think they're still licking their extensive wounds when they put me in the huge garbage can. My Bad?"

One week later Philly Raccoon went to see the physical therapist at the Montreal Neurological Institute and explained that Raccoons are supposed to have high foodies to exercise ratio, after which the physical therapist told him not to see a personal trainer, and gave him stick!

Philly is now using it to help him walk.
Question:
   18. **Why was it important for Philly to see a physical therapist?**

Philly Raccoon goes to the dentist
(This one's in described video for those
with impaired imagination)

Philly Raccoon is summoned every four months to go to the dentist in Hudson. Now you may think that after his experiences in hospital that he would cause trouble, but that is not the case, and here's why. Philly likes his hygienist, her name is Sara, she's from Iran, very beautiful, and she has friends in common like Farideh and Anahita. Moreover, Sara is especially nice to Philly. But for some reason the examination always starts in the same way:

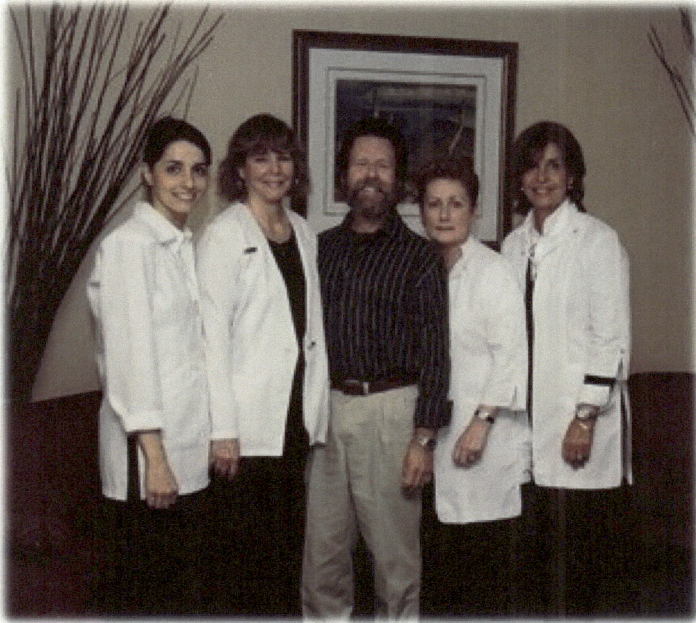

Sara: "Open wide"
Philly: "Ummm..." (Mouth firmly closed shut)

Sara: "Foodies!"
Philly: "Ahhh..."
Sara: (Very quickly turning her head away with gasping choking sounds as she says) "Have you been eating rotten fishy again?" (Reaching out for her gas mask)
Philly: "Arse"
Sara: "What did you say?" (Philly looking puzzled at the angry voice)
Philly: "Yarse!" (Said louder)
Sara: "That's better!" (Philly still looking puzzled)

Philly knows that having good sharp tooties is very good for raccoons, especially when practicing medicine (checking reflexes at the Montreal General Hospital). Although the cleaning does hurt a bit, he has learnt that staring into Sara's lovely brown eyes makes him think about good things, and besides she allows him to play with all the tools when she's not looking so he doesn't get bored (Philly likes playing dentist). The whole procedure takes about forty minutes to an hour including the interrogation; "**do you brush your tooties properly, and don't forget to floss**!" Then Philly Raccoon looks around for his presents; Sara gives him a tooties brush, tapered bushes to go on the end of a stick to chew on, and floss to play with (but this time not with the patients in the waiting room). He is then led outside to JoAnne the nice receptionist who tells him that it's covered by insurance. Philly always plays a joke on Sara by putting on his little "sad face", pointing to Sara accusingly, and saying at the top of his voice in the waiting room "She!.....Tortured me!". Then both Philly and Sara smile at each other, Philly showing of his nice shiny tooties (instilling fear in the waiting room) before going home.

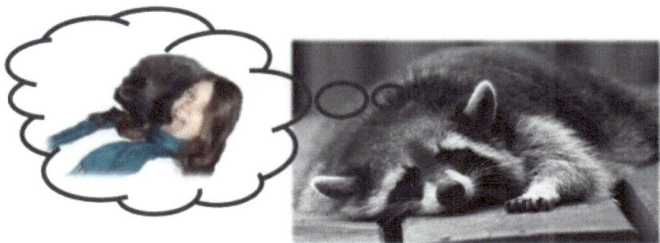

Philly Raccoon sometimes has dreams of being a dentist.

Question:

19. Why do you think it's important for Philly to make regular visits to the dentist?

Philly Raccoon goes for an audition

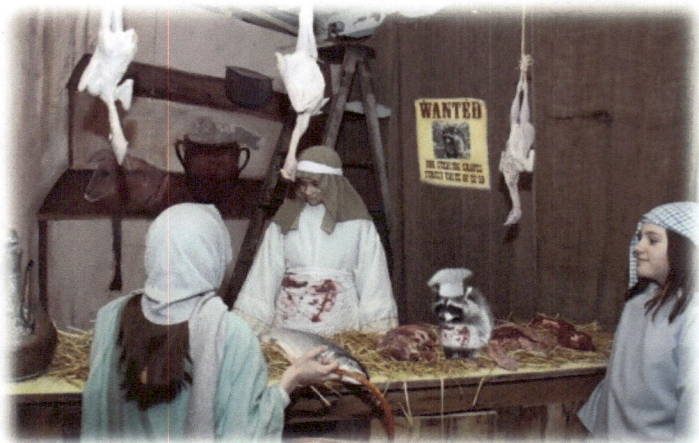

As everyone knows, raccoons like to act and show-off, and Philly was no exception. Hearing that there was a specific need and urgent prayer requests to get animals acting in the Walk to Bethlehem this year, Philly Raccoon arose to the occasion and turned up to the auditions to try his paw at acting. Because Philly likes foodies, he decided to try auditioning for the part in the market place as a server on the meat and fishy stall. Everything went well until the Director and everyone else noticed a poster on the wall of a raccoon wanted for stealing grapes with a street value of $2.50, who had a striking resemblance to that of Philly. He also blew his lines because he was distracted by the big fishy on the counter, and he couldn't concentrate on his part. As a result Philly failed the audition and had to try something else. Coincidentally, the big fishy also mysteriously disappeared from the market place.

Not being one for being put off, Philly then auditioned to be a singing angel. Philly being a very clever raccoon, he knows that intelligent people wear lots of different "hats" (each one having a particular role). His plan was set, he borrowed Rebecca's favorite brown (singing) hat with her permission while she wasn't looking, put it on his head, and posed like her to the best of his ability; he sang, and sang, and sang, figuring out that with all this careful preparation his voice has to come out good. It didn't work! Unfortunately for him, "Rotten fishy breath" took center stage, which was later identified to be the one from the counter. Philly then made a quick exit "Stage right".

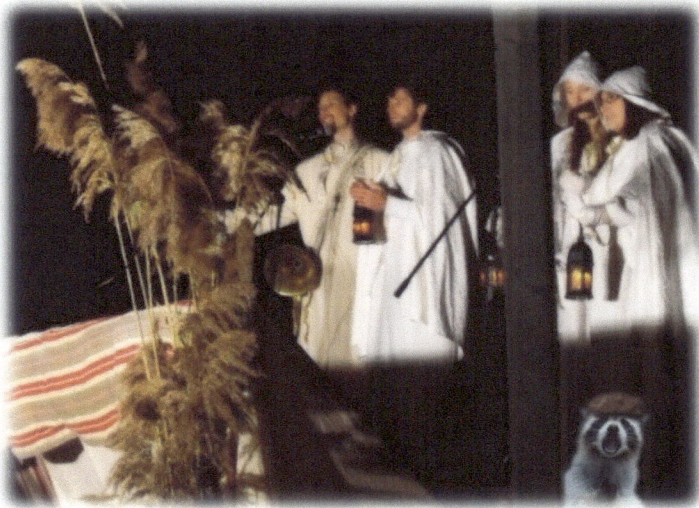

Philly Raccoon goes to the Walk to Bethlehem

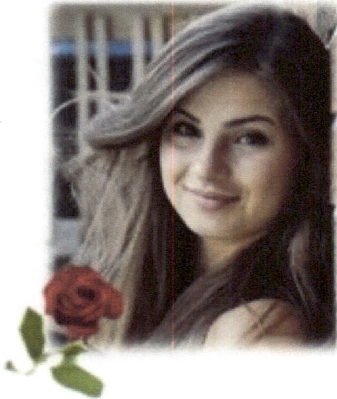

Philly Raccoon had heard a lot of good things about the Walk to Bethlehem and wanted to go, not only to see it and listen to the singing, but also to hear about Jesus Christ and get the bracelet with the beads that explains it. All this meant that Philly had to go into hibernation later that year. It was the last night and Philly turned up and joined a group. Everything went well and he behaved himself until he got to the market place, and then he saw all the foodies, eating all he could despite people trying to stop him. What he couldn't eat he held in his paws for later. A nice lady named Lea gave Philly a red rose, he didn't know it at the time, but that was to be the signal for the Romans to put him in prison; she's was a Roman Spy! The Romans did eventually catch him, confiscated his goodies and threw him in jail. It was the custom at the time for the Romans to make the rest of the group sing before the prisoner could be released. However, it was only after Philly started to sing that they opened the doors really wide to let him out before "rotten fishy breath" took hold.   Philly was captivated by the scene at the stable with Mary, Joseph, and baby Jesus; Philly Raccoon especially loved Rebecca's singing (notice that Rebecca's wearing her favorite brown hat).

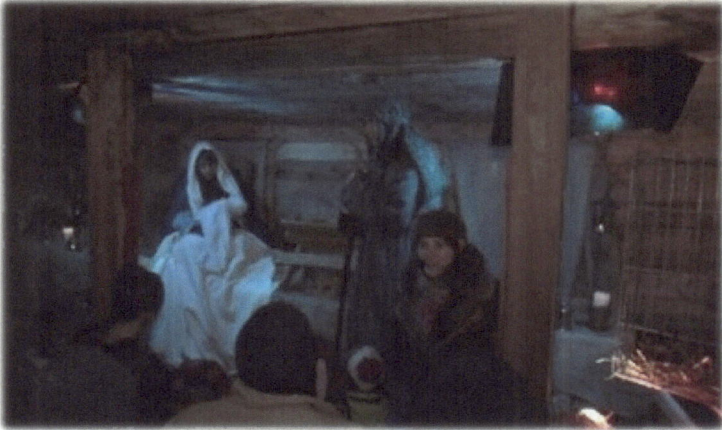

After the walk was over, Philly went to get his hot chocolate, foodies, and most important, his bead bracelet and to hear about Jesus at the welcome cafe. Being a little raccoon, Philly wasn't as welcomed as he had hoped, plus the fact that news got round of what he did in the market place.

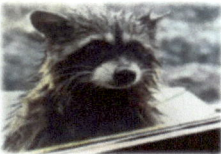

All he could do was look through the window. Feeling cold at this time he decided to warm himself by the fire at the Mary and Joseph scene before finding a place to hibernate. He eventually chose to be near the stable scene because he loves Rebecca's voice. He found a small hole in the ground under the stable and proceeded to dig. The ground was hard and his paws began to hurt but he knew he had to finish it. Philly Raccoon was so sad and heartbroken that he cried himself to sleep. Then an angel of the LORD came along side him gently stroking his head and said: "Listen! This is just a dream, but very clever raccoon's can hear dreams, so please, just listen", then Philly dreamt of his favorite bible story, that of the feeding of the five thousand (what else would a raccoon dream of). Philly traveled back in time to see the miracle take place. The disciples of Jesus said: "send the people away because they had no foodies", but Jesus said "No!" Then a boy came who had two fishes and five bread bits and offered these to Jesus. Jesus took the two fishes and five bread bits and giving thanks, started to give these out, the foodies didn't disappear, and he kept on giving them out. The disciples were distributing the food, and Philly asked one of them if he may have some please, the disciple said yes, and Philly said thank you. Philly enjoyed eating the foodies and wanted more. He thought that he would try to break it up in order to make more just like Jesus did, but he just ended up with fish bits and crumbs. He then went to see Jesus, got passed the disciples who were trying to protect him, Philly flung his paws round Him, and wouldn't let go despite their efforts to peel him off. Jesus told the disciples to leave Philly alone. Philly Raccoon was thinking "He knows my name!" Philly then took a step back and bowed out of respect and then looked into His eyes.

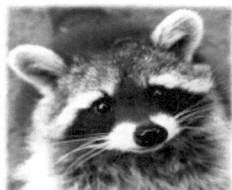

Jesus smiled and said "I have a gift especially for you". Philly was jumping up and down with excitement with his paws held high ready to receive the gift. Jesus then gave him a party bag full of goodies, Philly said thank you LORD (almost a whisper), he was overwhelmed, humbled, and very happy with his goodies, and then his dream ended with the sound of Rebecca's singing.

Philly's body was discovered the following day in a shallow grave (marked with a red rose). His blood soaked paws tightly holding onto a brown paper bag: containing a bracelet of colored beads, a fish sandwich, a small box of cheese nips, and a bar of chocolate.

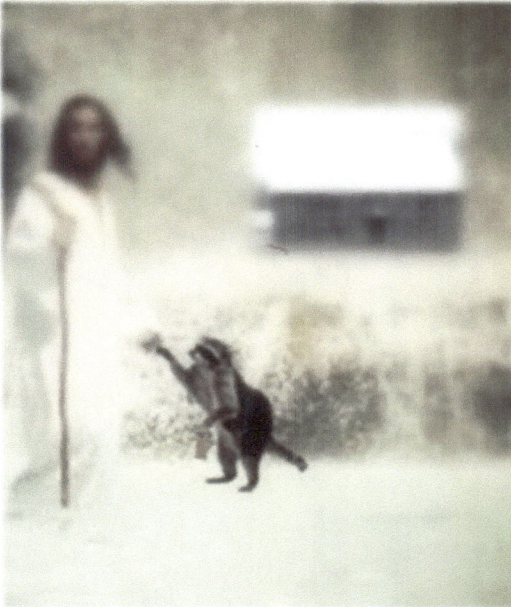

Your assignment just for fun:

Compile a full physiological profile of Philly Raccoon based upon all of these stories.

Answers to the questions

1. **F.A.S.T.** is an easy way to remember the sudden signs of a stroke. Helen should have done these simple actions that could save a life:

   a. **Face Drooping** – Helen should have asked Philly to smile, looking out for an uneven smile or face drooping.

   b. **Arm (Paw) Weakness** – Helen should have asked Philly to raise both paws, and see if one paw drifts downward.

   c. **Speech Difficulty** – Philly should have been asked some simple questions (in Philly's case very simple).

   d. **Time to call the emergency services** – If Philly had any of these symptoms, even if the symptoms were to go away, the emergency services must be called and he should be taken to hospital immediately. Make a note of the time when the first symptoms appeared, as this would be very useful for the medical staff to know when they take the patients history.

2. Anti-Nuclear Antibodies (ANAs) was normal indicating that Philly's condition was not autoimmune in nature. Vitamin B12 levels were surprisingly high. Low levels of vitamin B12 are

associated with ataxia. High levels can be associated with liver cirrhosis, hepatitis, polycythemia vera or myelocytic leukemia, which was not the case. However, Philly suggested that a high level of vitamin B12 could indicate the presence of anti-vitamin B12 antibodies able to effectively increase the half-life of the vitamin, and at the same time eliminating its function, hence causing the ataxia. Although Philly mentioned this to the doctors nothing came of it. What do you think of Philly's idea?

3. The word "**Ataxia**" comes from the Greek meaning "**lack of order**" the symptoms in Philly's case indicated cerebella ataxia and is used to indicate ataxia that is due to dysfunction of the cerebellum. Ataxia is not a diagnosis but is a description of the symptoms. Possible causes of ataxia are as follows and this is not a definitive list:

   a. Stroke

   b. Brain tumor

   c. Multiple sclerosis

   d. Parkinson's disease

   e. Exogenous substances, such as occurs with chronic ethanol consumption, and one for Philly to note, that of methylmercury through consumption of fishy with high mercury concentrations.

f. Vitamin B12 deficiency

g. Wilson's disease

h. Gluten ataxia

i. Hereditary ataxia's

j. Lyme's disease

k. Vitamin E deficiency

l. Creutzfeldt–Jakob disease (CJD)

4. Most people as well as Philly Raccoon have experienced doctors tapping their knees with a rubber hammer (Philly didn't like it). The normal response is a 'knee jerk', and is an example of a reflex, which is an involuntary muscular response, elicited by the rubber hammer tapping the associated tendon. When a reflex response is abnormal, it may be due to the disruption of the sensory (feeling) or motor (movement) nerves or both. To determine where the neurological problem may be, the doctor will test reflexes in different parts of the body.

5. *Dystonia* is a disorder characterized by involuntary muscle contractions that cause slow repetitive movements or abnormal postures. Philly thinks he's got "**focal dystonia**" that affects a muscle only on his right paw causing an abnormal posture, when he's not thinking, which happens rather a lot.

6. **(a & d)** The CBC with peripheral smear along with the ESR would give an overall picture as to whether or not a mini stroke may have been the root cause of the ataxia. In addition granules in the basophiles may be an indication of lead poisoning, the symptoms of which also include ataxia.

(c & g) The ceruloplasmin level along with the 24hr urinary copper was assessed to determine whether or not Philly had Wilson's disease. Wilson's disease is an autosomal recessive genetic disorder in which copper accumulates in tissues manifesting itself as neurological and/or psychiatric symptoms, and liver disease. In Wilson's disease, the plasma ceruloplasmin concentration would be lower than normal (<0.2 g/L), and urinary copper concentrations would be high (>50 μg/24h).

(b) ALT levels are indicative of parenchymal liver cell damage, which occurs not only in Wilson's disease (see above), but it's also abnormally raised in cases of chronic ethanol abuse, which is also a possible cause of ataxia.

(e) Vitamin E deficiency results in poor conduction of electrical impulses along nerves manifesting itself as ataxia.

(f) Anti-cardiolipin antibodies (ACAs) are antibodies against cardiolipin and found in a variety diseases, including syphilis. The later stages of syphilis results in neurological damage and symptoms including ataxia. Philly was most embarrassed, but it did turn out to be negative.

7. The consultant suggested that Philly was crossed-wired. Difficult for Philly Raccoon to know for sure why the consultant said that, but perhaps she thought that Philly had a mini stroke, or that it was just psychological.

8. Can stress be responsible for Philly Raccoon's symptoms? In the absence of other symptoms Philly thinks it's very unlikely. In addition, the ataxia observed was progressive and not intermittent, which is not indicative of a stress related cause.

9. Was the consultant right in saying that Philly ort to see a personal trainer? Definitely not, however, she must have had a change of heart in the end, because she did book Philly to see the physical therapist at the Montreal Neurological Institute. Good choice!

10. What was on Philly's mind when he asked for a "14-3-3 test" and an "electroencephalogram" (EEG)? Detectable 14-3-3 protein in the cerebrospinal fluid (CSF) is indicative of substantial and relatively rapid neuronal destruction. Increased CSF concentrations of 14-3-3 proteins have been described in patients with various forms of Creutzfeldt-Jakob disease (CJD), more specifically Philly was thinking about "MV or VV

type2" in which cerebellum symptoms i.e. ataxia predominate. Obviously the prognosis is not good; showing the "Dark Side" of Philly's thinking. The EEG may be used in conjunction looking for characteristic abnormal waves, which would not be the case if it was "MV or VV type 2". Philly should have really done his homework on that one. Philly also couldn't understand why the consultant assumed that a 14-3-3 result would come back as a false positive.

11. The consultant probably thinks he's had a mini stroke and that the condition is not progressive. Alternatively she may be thinking that it's purely psychological. Philly doesn't think it's psychological, because when there's a parcel of goodies up stairs and he wants to get to it quickly before it goes away, without even thinking he runs all zombie like, must be funny to watch!

12. Philly can only think that this black list is either one given to insurance companies so you can't get life insurance; or if it is positive, one would have to diagnose Philly as having possible CJD. An investigation would have to be initiated to determine possible causes. Philly would be more embarrassed if people knew he was tested for ACAs, how would he explain that one to people at Church?

13. The list so far of what Philly thinks he hasn't got:

a. Stroke

b. Brain tumor

c. Multiple sclerosis

d. Parkinson's disease

e. Exogenous substances, such as occurs with chronic ethanol consumption, and one for Philly to note, that of methylmercury through consumption of fishy with high mercury concentrations (Philly says that he only gets his fishy from the best garbage cans)

f. Vitamin B12 deficiency (Philly is still thinking of his idea)

g. Wilson's disease

h. Gluten ataxia (Philly's not ruling it out completely)

i. Hereditary ataxia's (no family history and Philly's twin brother has not shown any symptoms to date)

j. Lyme's disease

k. Vitamin E deficiency

14. Philly's previous MRI was only 6 Months ago, and at first glance one might say that it wasn't a

good call, but note that the previous MRI did not include prior IV administration of Gadolinium.

15. Philly wasn't actually injected with the metal itself, but a chelate of Gadolinium "Gd(III)" which does not pass through the blood–brain barrier because it's hydrophilic. Thus, these are useful in enhancing lesions following a stoke, and tumors where the Gd(III) leaks out. Because the metal is paramagnetic it works by shortening the T1 relaxation time of protons located nearby, and thus enhancing the image.

16. The consultant wanted to know if the blood brain barrier was compromised, hence the purpose of performing the MRI. Although such lesions should have been picked up on the first MRI, the use of the Gadolinium (III) chelate ensures that nothing would be overlooked.

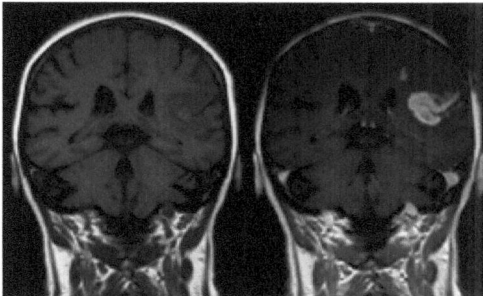

Effect of contrast agent on images: Defect of the blood–brain barrier after stroke shown in MRI. T_1-weighted images, left image without, right image with the contrast medium administration. **(Philly wanted to make it clear that this is not his brain).**

17. It is very important to assess the patient's kidney function before administering gadolinium contrast agents. A rare but serious side effect in patients with renal failure known as Nephrogenic Systemic Fibrosis (NSF) associated with exposure to gadolinium that involves fibrosis of skin, joints, eyes, and internal organs. The cause is not fully understood and there is no known cure. (We heard that Philly gave the laboratory staff lots of wee wee, so his kidneys were assumed to have been working properly).

18. It was important for Philly to see a physical therapist because that person would have been trained and licensed to examine, evaluate, diagnose and treat impairment, functional limitations and disabilities in patients. Definitely not to be confused with a personal trainer (especially the "no gain without pain" ones). The physical therapist Philly went to see was Caroline, and she specifically specializes in neurology.

19. Philly knows that regular dental visits are important because they help keep your tooties and tootie holders (gums) healthy. But what he didn't know is that there's a strong relationship between your oral health and your overall health, so taking good care of your mouth is a big part of taking care of your whole body.

Bacteria from untreated gum disease can actually spread infection to other parts of your body. In the case of bacterial endocarditis, this affects the inner lining of the heart and the surfaces of its valves. The bacteria stick to these surfaces and create growths or pockets of bacteria and make you sick.

The BSE outbreak in the UK and cases of Creutzfeldt–Jakob disease observed now

For the first time in the UK, Bovine spongiform encephalopathy (BSE) [1] was officially recognized in cattle 1986, although there was evidence that it could have been picked up earlier in 1984. It was assumed that this had originated from the scrapie agent, which had been present in sheep in the United Kingdom for over 200 years, and that the scrapie agent jumped species when sheep offal was included in protein supplements and fed to cattle. After the cattle started to die, cattle carcasses and offal were included in the same protein supplements thus adding to the epidemic.

The epidemic in cattle in Britain reached incredible proportions; by 1993 more than 1,000 cases per week were being reported, not to mention wide-spread panic. The problem was traced to feed supplements containing infected cow and sheep parts. In the early 1980s there was a change to the rendering process by which livestock carcasses are converted to various products, including protein supplements for livestock feed. Previously, a solvent extraction step had been used to extract fats. However, this step was omitted when the price of the petroleum-based solvents used to extract fats went up. The infectious agent being solvent-sensitive was then permitted to be incorporated into the livestock feed. Although protein supplements containing sheep and cattle offal were banned in the UK in 1988, it was not until 1991-1992 that this ban was strictly enforced. Given the long incubation of BSE, the epidemic curve didn't start going downward until late 1993.

BSE Cases in the UK during 1988 until 2012 [1,2]

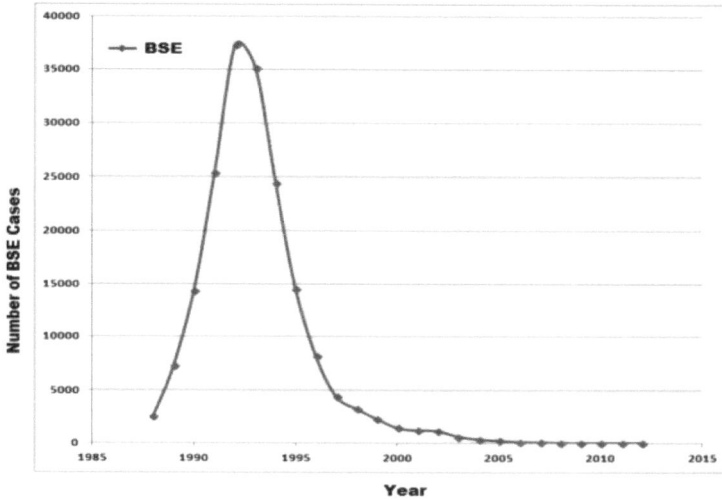

On March 21, 1996 it went public that 10 cases of CJD (later referred to as variant or vCJD) in people not otherwise considered high risk. These individuals were much younger with an average age of 27 as opposed to 63 that occur sporadically (sporadic or sCJD) everywhere in the world at an incidence of about one per million per year. I remember being at a clinical biochemistry conference eating a rare beef sandwich at an evening reception when the news was announced. My only course of action at the time was to wash it down with a pint of beer. Seriously, the disease in this age group, associated with symptoms and duration that had never been seen before. Therefore, one has to conclude that this is a new disease and not your typical CJD, and may well be linked to the species (i.e. bovine or sheep) from which the individual has been infected.

BSE Cases along with vCJD in the UK during 1988 until 2012 [1,2,3]

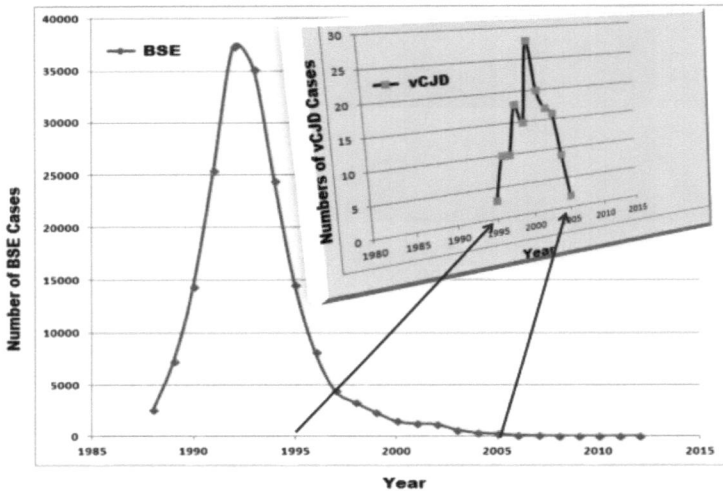

Although very tragic and still is, the cases of vCJD related to the BSE outbreak was fortunately extremely small considering the number of people who would have consumed the contaminated beef products. As we will discover later, this is only part of the full story. Cases of sCJD still outnumbered those of vCJD during the same period of time, but the trend seems to be increasing? Looking at the graph above, we are probably talking about a 7 to 10 year incubation period from the time that the beef was first consumed until the disease was recognised. In other words the average age of the people when the beef products were consumed would have been around 17.

Deaths of Patients with Definite of Probable CJD in the UK [3]

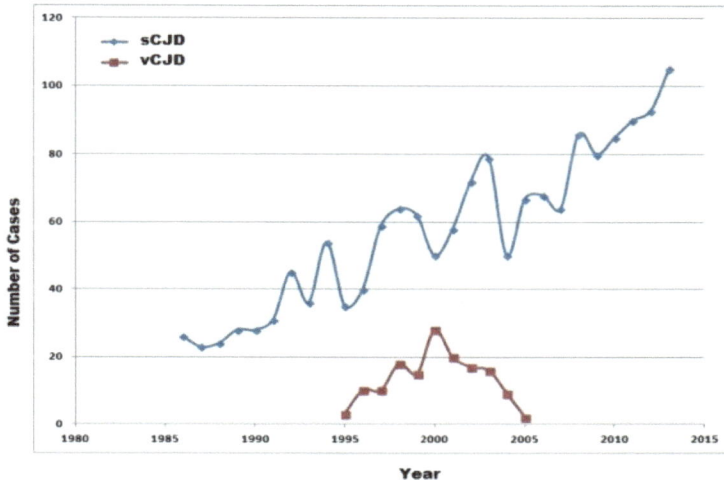

Now why is the trend increasing? Well first of all we have to know something about the nature of the causative agent and the pathogenesis of the disease.

It was Dr. Stanley Prusiner of the University of California, San Francisco who first elucidated the nature of the causative agent of BSE and its human equivalent CJD [2]. In recognition of his work he received the Nobel Prize in Physiology or Medicine in 1997. The causative agent itself was like no other discovered. It was not a virus or a super tough bacterium because it contained no nucleic acids (DNA or RNA), but ended up to be a protein to which he coined the term "prion (PrP)" to denote a protein infectious agent. These proteins have about 250 amino acids and are in fact abnormal variants of the normal protein (PrP^c) present in normal cells such as brain cells. The differences between the normal (PrP^c) and abnormal prions (PrP) do not lie in their primary structure (the sequence of their amino acids), but rather in their folding (secondary structure). The secondary structure of a normal prion predominantly adopts a α-helical configuration whereas the abnormal prion mainly consists of β-pleated sheets. The pathogenesis of the disease is even more bizarre; when the abnormal prions enter the body, they are able to convert their normal counterparts into more of the abnormal forms. Presumably the proteins go from a high to a lower energy state hence why they do not readily convert back. Furthermore, the abnormal prion is resistant to protease degradation so that overtime there is a build up of PrP aggregates, especially in neurons in the brain. It is this aggregation of PrP around and in the neurons that are responsible for the pathology; brain cells die accounting for the progressive symptoms.

I had to explain it to Philly Raccoon like this; it's like the zombie apocalypse but at the molecular level. Philly is still very scared at the prospect of turning into a zombie raccoon. I think enough said.

Methionine - Valine (M-V) Polymorphism
As I mentioned before, the PrP has a normal counterpart PrP^c, and there are genetic variations of this normal counterpart, the main one being at codon 129 which either codes for methionine "M" or valine "V". Each one of us has two copies of the gene (one from each parent). So either we could be "MM", "MV", or "VV". Although this polymorphism does not cause the disease in itself, it does account for the wide range of symptoms and perhaps the susceptibility observed in individuals affected with CJD [4].

A. M-V Polymorphism in the general population

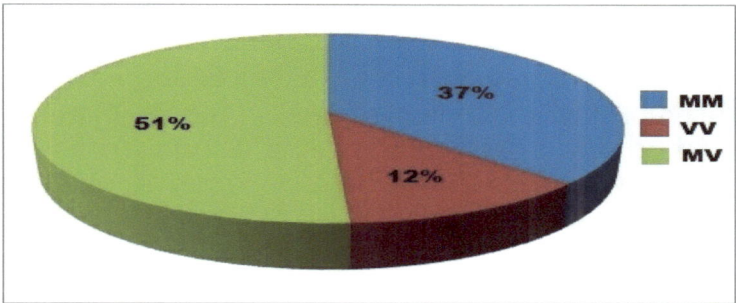

B. Sporadic CJD

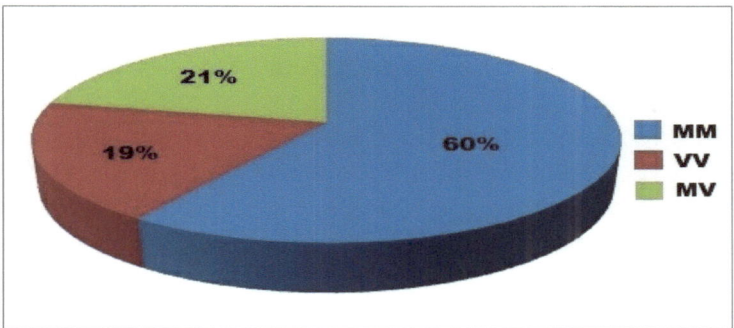

C. Variant CJD

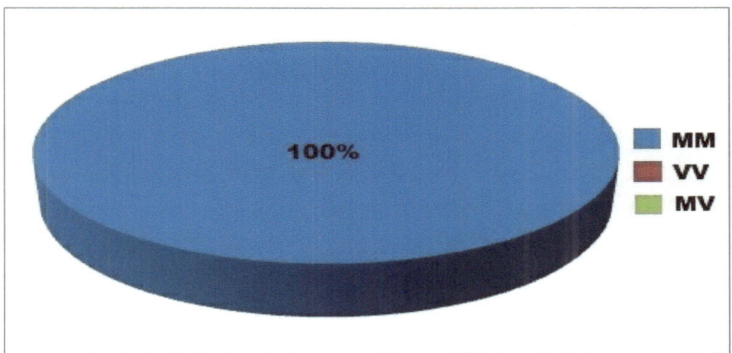

Now we have our first lead as to what might have been going on during the BSE outbreak. Notice that all of the CJD cases that were attributed to the consumption of contaminated beef products classified as vCJD were all of the "MM" genotype, which only comprises of 37% of the total population. If we also take into account that these people would have been in their teens when they consumed the contaminated beef products, this 37% would go down even further. It is also interesting to note that in sCJD the "MM" genotype also is disproportionately higher.

What Happened during the BSE Outbreak?
The general population not just the "MM" genotype must have consumed the contaminated beef products. What if the incubation period for the abnormal beef generated prion to cause disease in people of the "MM" genotype is between 7 to 10 years. We see a number of cases in younger people average age of 27 years, but they were exposed to the infectious agent approximately ten years previously. Now consider people who were of the "MM" genotype and were exposed to the infectious agent from say 30 years old onwards. The disease would obviously manifest itself later in life and get misclassified as sCJD, because now we are talking about an older age group.

From the graph on the following page, prior to the initial outbreak of vCJD, 1970 to 1994 (blue and red lines) spanning a period of 25 years, not much happened. However, from 1995 until 2004 the time period for which the vCJD cases appeared (green line) there was a huge jump of sCJD cases over that same period of time, and it would not be unreasonable to assume that these additional numbers were people of the "MM" genotype who acquired the disease when they were older. It doesn't stop there, the numbers are still increasing 2005 to 2013 (purple line). Now it would be said that the numbers are increasing because we are now better at diagnosing the disease. I would like to put that aside for a moment and come up with an alternative hypothesis.

Prediction of more cases of CJD as a result of eating contaminated beef during the 80's and beyond, misclassified as sCJD [5]

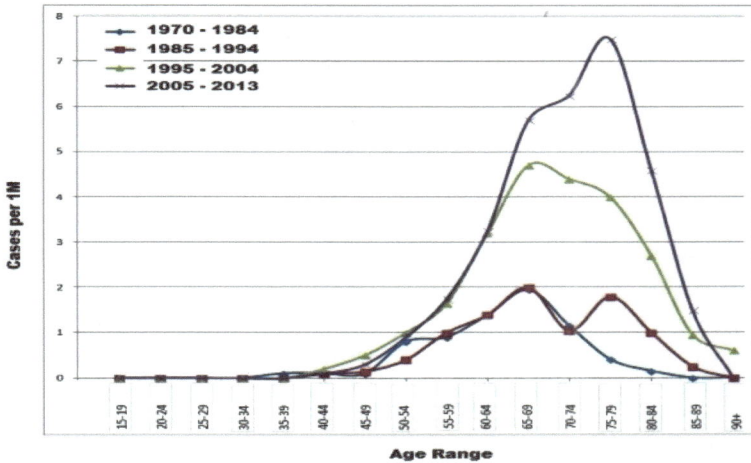

As we have seen above, people with the "MV" and "VV" genotype also get sCJD. If we assume that the abnormal prion from beef also produces the disease in people who are "MV" or "VV" genotypes, one would expect the incubation period to be extended based upon the initial vCJD cases. Therefore, I'm not surprised that these numbers are on the increase. If we wait long enough we may actually find the numbers going down to those observed in 1970 to 1994, which I would consider as baseline. It would be interesting to see how these figures from the UK compare with other countries.

Why does CJD have a Wide Range of Symptoms?
Dr. Pierluigi Gambettia and his team at the National Prion Disease Pathology Surveillance Center Case

Western Reserve University managed to answer this question by collating the polymorphism at codon 129 of the individual (i.e. MM, MV, or VV), and the break down fragment of the abnormal prion following treatment with the enzyme proteinase K [4] . Within a particular individual either the PrP is broken down up to amino acid 82, or up amino acid 97 from the N-terminus, denoted as fragments 1 and 2, respectively when the PrP is treated with the enzyme. So there are six possibilities: MM-1, MM-2, MV-1, MV-2, VV-1, and VV-2. Subsequently, when the symptoms of 300 individuals were collated in 1999, the classification of sCJD based upon molecular and genotypic analysis was established, and it made perfect sense. However, these experiments and observations would have been done with the scapie agent (PrP^{sc}). What if the abnormal prion from cattle is different, it may account for a whole new set of symptoms, some of which may not have been observed before?

In a BBC News article published in 2004 entitled BSE link to different CJD types [6] it states:
"Eating BSE-infected meat could lead to people developing different types of CJD, researchers have suggested. Until now, it had been thought that BSE was only linked to the variant form of Creutzfeldt - Jakob disease, but Medical Research Council experts say BSE may also manifest itself as sporadic CJD, or a new form of the disease not yet seen in humans. The study, in Science, raises the possibility that more people than previously thought may be at risk."

So what can be done?
I think a good sound scientific approach is needed; let us aim to make the word "sporadic" a thing of the past,

by that I mean a full investigation should be carried out for each and every patient. First get a genotype for the normal prion, providing it doesn't cause harm to the patient, second and most important is to get a biopsy of the lymphoid tissue of the tonsil and stain it for the abnormal prions. Should this test be positive, then one can conclude that the transmission of the disease was by the consumption of contaminated food, which would be very useful to know, and to investigate further. A full history should be taken to look for a genetic and/or even a life-style link. In addition, I would also like to see the biopsy of the tonsil test done on patients with Alzheimer's just to see if ingested abnormal prions may be responsible for this devastating disease. I suppose I'm wondering if there could be a possibility of a misdiagnosis, mistaking CJD for Alzheimer's which appears to be on the increase.

Philly being a very clever raccoon came up with an idea for a possible cure; for which he's hoping to get the prestigious "Big Plate Foodies Prize" for Physiology or Medicine. For this to really work one really needs to understand at a molecular level the interactions between the PrP (PrP^{sc} / PrP^{bse}) and PrP^c and how the conversion takes place. Having established the mode of action one can develop an "aptamer" to bind to the appropriate part of the abnormal prion thus inactivating it, in its tracks. Not only would this approach be useful for CJD, but also for Alzheimer's, and any other disease associated with abnormal prions.

To this end I will be sending out letters on behalf of Philly Raccoon with details of the proposal to some leading scientists that I can think of along with a copy of this book as an encouragement, after all he does deserve a big plate of foodies.

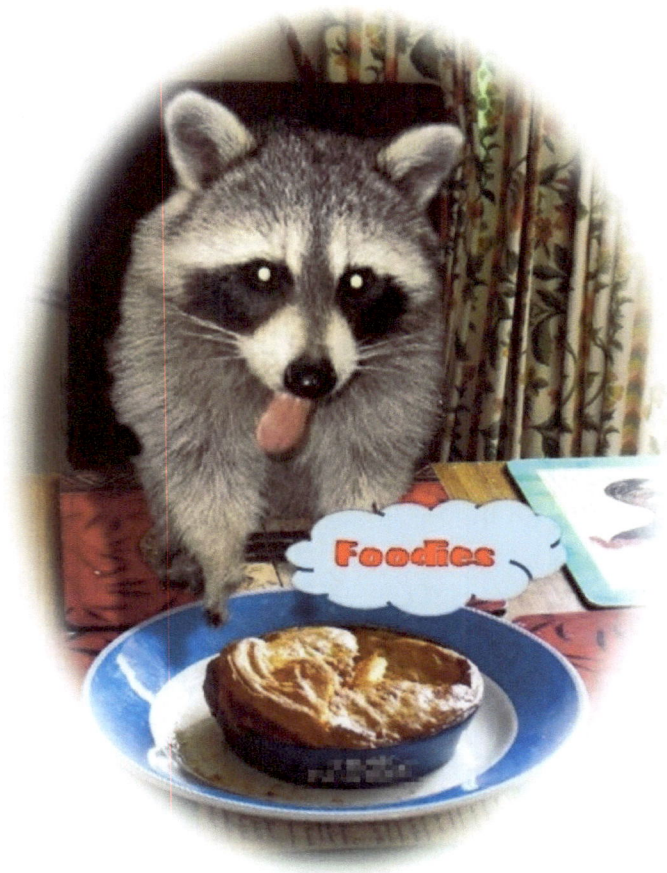

Foodies

References and background reading

1. World Health Organization.
WHO manual for surveillance of human transmissible spongiform encephalopathies, including vCJD.
ISBN 92 4 154588 7

2. Prion Disease and the BSE Crisis
Stanley B. Prusiner
Science 10 October 1997: Vol. 278 no. 5336 pp. 245-251
http://www.sciencemag.org/site/feature/data/prusiner/245.xhtml

3. CJD in the UK (by calendar year)
The National CJD Research & Surveillance Unit, Western General Hospital, Edinburgh, EH4 2XU
http://www.cjd.ed.ac.uk/documents/figs.pdf

4. Mechanisms of phenotypic heterogeneity in prion, Alzheimer and other conformational diseases
Pierluigi Gambettia, Piero Parchib, Sabina Capellarib, Claudio Russoc, Massimo Tabatonc, Jan K. Tellerd and Shu G. Chena
Journal of Alzheimer's Disease 3 (2001) 87–95
ISSN 1387-2877

5. 22nd Annual Report 2013 CJD Surveillance in the UK. The National CJD Research & Surveillance Unit, Western General Hospital, Edinburgh, EH4 2XU
http://www.cjd.ed.ac.uk/documents/report22.pdf

6. BBC NEWS (Report issued in 2004)
BSE 'link to different CJD types'
http://news.bbc.co.uk/2/hi/health/4003789.stm